Midwifery Care and the Growing Home Birth Movement in Kentucky

ASHLI FINDLEY

ISBN: 978-0-9998831-3-6 (Paperback)
ISBN: 978-0-9998831-4-3 (e-book)

Cover image by Katie Lacer/MommaKTShoots.
Book design by Pryor Graphics & Designs, LLC.

Printed in the United States of America.

First printing December 9, 2019.

Contents

Preface

While the United States is facing a maternal mortality crisis, the outcomes for Kentucky mothers is not any better. A full 35.1% of Kentucky mothers deliver by Cesarean section, while the national average is 32.2%. A total 10.7% of babies are born premature versus the national rate of 9.6%. Only 8.6% of births are vaginal birth after Cesarean (VBAC) compared to the 11.3% national average. And the list goes on.

With these dire statistics, the home birth movement continues to grow. Women are choosing to take control of where they birth, how they give birth, and who their birth attendant is. Home births in the U.S. have increased, on average, 4.50% every year since 2004. In Kentucky, that figure is 6.40%.

In 1988, the overall home birth rate in Kentucky was 0.35%. Fast forward to 2016, that percentage was 1.35%. That's almost a four-fold increase. That's also more growth than home births happening nationwide. Today, just shy of 1% of U.S. births happen at home, which is also an increase – from 0.56% in 2004.

Over 700 births (and counting) are happening at home every year in Kentucky. These figures may seem small, but they do represent a trend in where women are choosing to give birth.

For those women choosing to birth at home, the care providers who are helping to deliver these babies are largely certified professional midwives (CPMs), mother-centered professionals who view birth as a natural occurrence rather than a medical event.

The irony? CPMs in Kentucky only recently won legislation in March 2019 that will now grant them the legal licensure to practice – something that has not been granted since 1975. The win is big news, as the outcomes for mothers of CPM-attended births include: fewer drugs and medical interventions, lower costs, fewer low birth weight infants, lower rates of infection, stronger parent–infant bonding, higher rates of breastfeeding, and greater satisfaction for women and families.

What women nationwide, and in Kentucky, are really saying is, "We know our bodies. We know what quality care looks like. We want mother-centered care. And we are willing to leave hospitals in search of it."

This is that story. This is that education. This publication highlights evidence-based data on home birth and midwifery care. Some sections highlight the role that current health care professionals play in this environment of increasing home births, and other sections highlight the legal ramifications of this new bill that legislators have put in place.

The end goal is a comprehensive publication that provides solid information and research to help improve Kentucky's maternal and newborn care and mortality rates.

Let's get started.

Section I: Introduction: Where We're at as a Country

In order to understand the continuing increase in home births in Kentucky, under the care of midwives, it's important to look at what's going on in the background...

A Nationwide Crisis

It is now well-documented that the United States is the most dangerous developed nation in the world to give birth. Alison Young of USA Today highlighted this in her popular piece "Hospitals know how to protect mothers. They just aren't doing it" when she wrote, "...the U.S. continues to watch other countries improve as it falls behind."[1]

Why?

According to her piece, "women needlessly die and suffer life-changing injuries in childbirth because medical staff aren't following long-known safety measures." These are standard, low-tech safety procedures like weighing bloody pads to track blood loss as a way to monitor the danger of a new mother bleeding internally until her organs shut down; or giving medication within an hour of spotting high blood pressure to reduce the incidence of having a stroke.

For those new mothers who don't die, some are left paralyzed. Some have to undergo emergency hysterectomies (whether they are appropriately informed of it or not), ensuring they are unable to have any more children. You can read the stories of some of these women in their own words at 50k.usatoday.com.

The odds are worse for black women, who are three to four times more likely to die of pregnancy- or childbirth-related complications than white

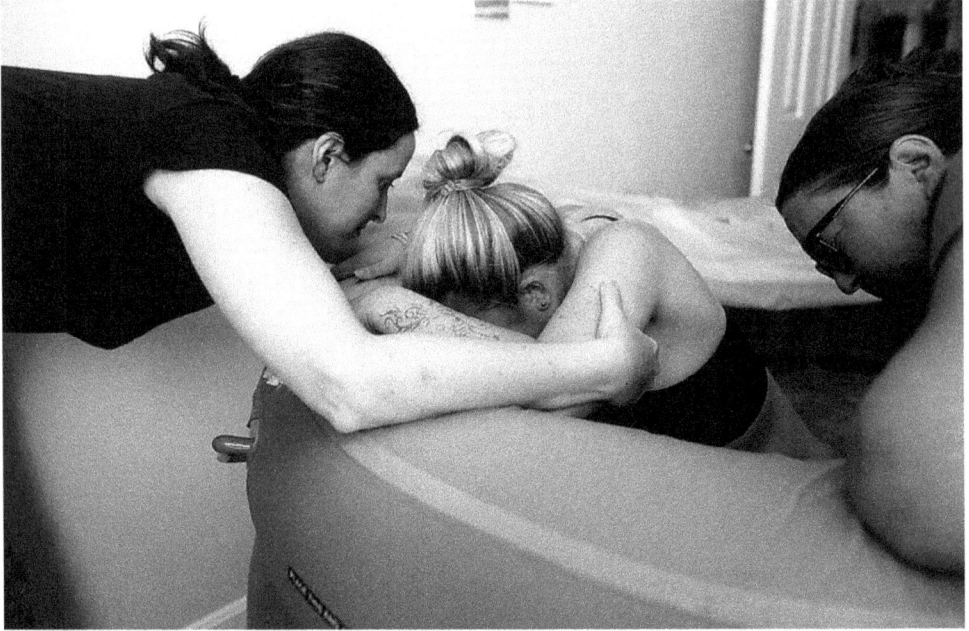

women. Not only has it been well documented that they face these same medical malpractices as white women, but they also endure systemic racism throughout the process – from their prenatal appointments with their OB and on-site nurse to when they show up at the hospital to give birth to postpartum care.

USA Today isn't the only major news outlet to uncover these truths. NPR, The New York Times, The Washington Post, and ProPublica have as well, just to name a few. For these primary reasons, and more, women are choosing to take back their autonomy and voice over their own bodies on how they give birth. More on that later.

Maternal Mortality and Morbidity

Maternal mortality or maternal death is defined as "a death that occurs to a woman as a direct result of obstetric complications or indirectly as a result of pregnancy-induced exacerbation of pre-existing medical conditions, but not as a result of incidental or accidental causes."[2] The World Health Organization (WHO) documents this as the death of a women while pregnant or within 42 days of termination of pregnancy.[3]

The major complications that account for nearly 75% of all maternal deaths are:

- Severe bleeding (mostly bleeding after childbirth)
- Infections (usually after childbirth)
- High blood pressure during pregnancy (pre-eclampsia and eclampsia)
- Complications from delivery
- Unsafe abortion

Futhermore, the WHO notes that "Most maternal deaths are preventable, as the healthcare solutions to prevent or manage complications are well known." For example, the risk of severe bleeding can be reduced by injecting Pitocin immediately after childbirth, and infection after childbirth can be eliminated if good hygiene is practiced and if early signs of infection are recognized and treated in a timely manner.

From 1990 to 2015, maternal deaths per 100,000 births in most developed nations has been flat or dropping. As of 2015, countries like Germany and Portugal had an average 9.0 maternal deaths per 100,000 live births. France had 7.8, Canada had 7.3, and Finland had 3.8. The U.S.? It rose from 16.9 in 1990 to 17.6 in 2000 to 26.4 in 2016.[4]

It is important to note that there is some controversy on how maternal mortality is measured in the U.S. versus much of the rest of the world. While the WHO documents death within 42 days, the U.S. has, in more recent history, used a measurement of death within one year.

U.S. data used for national and international comparisons are based on information reported on death certificates filed in state vital statistics offices, and subsequently compiled into national data through the National Vital Statistics System.

A pregnancy question was added to the U.S. standard death certificate in 2003 to improve verification of maternal deaths. The question has several checkboxes asking whether the female who died was: not pregnant within past year; pregnant at time of death; not pregnant, but pregnant within 42 days of death; not pregnant, but pregnant 43 days to 1 year before death; or unknown if pregnant within the past year.[5] There were delays in states' adoption of the revised death certificate and, thus, the new pregnancy question.[6][7]

As of January 1, 2014, however, all states except California, Colorado, Massachusetts, Virginia, and West Virginia were supplying pregnancy data for the standard 42-day timeframe.

A study was published in 2016 in an effort to provide an overview of U.S. maternal mortality trends from 2000–2014.[8] Simply totaling raw, unadjusted data from all states regardless of whether or not they revised their death certificates resulted in a reported U.S. maternal mortality rate that more than doubled from 9.8 maternal deaths per 100,000 live births in 2000 to 21.5 in 2014. Excluding data from California and Texas, the researchers provided an estimated maternal mortality rate from 2000–2014. That rate in 2000 was 18.8, and the rate increased to 23.8 in 2014 – an increase of 26.6%.

As mentioned earlier, aside from deaths, more than 50,000 women in the U.S. suffer serious and life-threatening complications from pregnancy and childbirth every year known as severe maternal morbidity.[9] That's the highest number in all of developed nations, and the only nation where that statistic has trended upwards in the last 20 years. The best estimates say half of those deaths could be prevented and half the injuries reduced or eliminated with better care.

Based on the rate per 10,000 deliveries, serious complications more than doubled from 1993 to 2014, driven largely by a five-fold rise in blood transfusions.[10] That also includes a nearly 60 percent rise in emergency hysterectomies; in 2014 alone, more than 4,000 women had emergency hysterectomies. The rates of new mothers requiring breathing tubes and of treatment for sepsis — a life-threatening inflammatory response to infection that can damage tissues and organs — both increased by 75%.

None of these estimates begins to include the other very real costs borne by women and families — psychological trauma and treatment, lost wages and long-term health effects.[11]

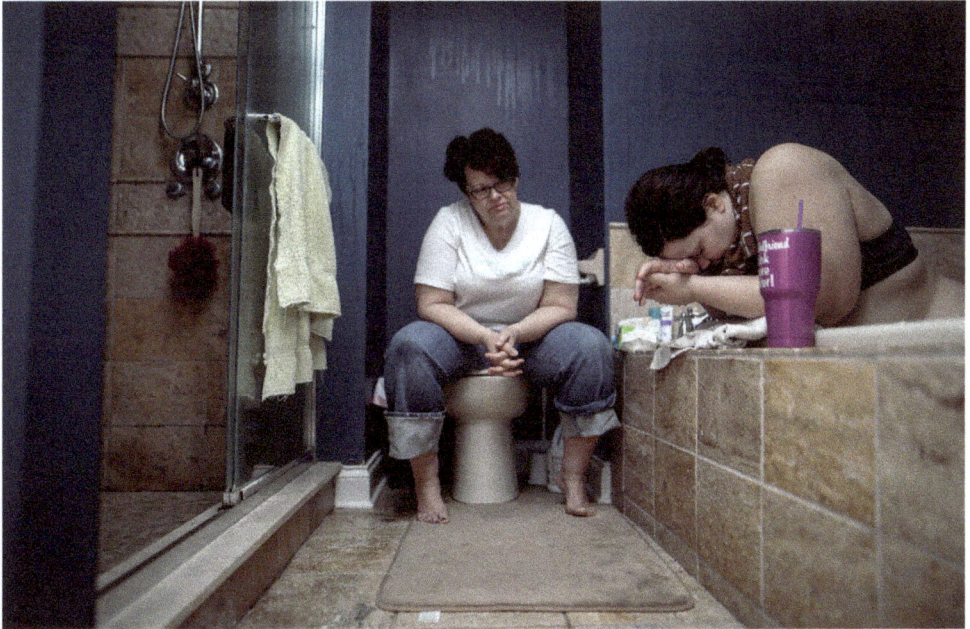

Copyright © 2018 Katie Lacer/MommaKTShoots

Obstetric Violence & Informed Consent

It's also important to note the increased commentary around "obstetric violence," a range of abusive actions taken upon women during labor – from nonconsensual episiotomies to outright sexual assault.[12]

The American College of Gynecologists and Obstetricians (ACOG) issued a comprehensive committee opinion affirming that a "decisionally capable" pregnant woman has the right to refuse treatment, and discouraging "in the strongest possible terms" the use of "duress, manipulation, coercion, physical force, or threats… to motivate women toward a specific clinical decision."[13]

Ananda Lowe's article, "A doula's call for a 'culture of consent' during childbirth," highlights the need for appropriate informed consent between provider and patient during childbirth, as well as a look at procedures that should create conversation for change,[14] like:

- Having a mother lie on her back to push the baby out, which makes vaginal delivery more difficult because gravity is working against her and the pelvis is more restricted than birthing standing up or on allfours [15];

- Being hooked up to continuous fetal monitoring. A 2006 review of three decades' worth of data found that it offered very little benefit for the majority of births and was actually associated with a higher rate of C-sections and vaginal deliveries with forceps[16];

- Forbidding women from eating and drinking during labor, which causes emotional stress, slightly longer labors, and less-nourished mothers[17] [18];

- Not allowing laboring women to change positions and move around freely, which has been shown to make birth more painful and difficult[19]

These actions breed a culture in America that showcases why almost one in four mothers said they did not fully understand that they had the legal right to clear and full explanations of any procedure during childbirth, and that they had the right to accept or refuse any procedure.

Lowe notes that a first step toward creating a culture of consent in maternity care would involve adding one simple sentence to many conversations. If a physician says, "I'm here to give you a vaginal exam," they can follow that by saying, "You have the right to say yes or no." That simple sentence embodies the spirit and the critical importance of informed consent in any area of health care, even in a crisis situation.

The goal is not to put sole blame doctors and nurses who fall short in these areas but, rather, to bring to the forefront of the public's attention to the tragedies that are happening so that we can get to work on the real solutions.

So, how does Kentucky compare?

The Birth Place Lab, a Division of Midwifery at the University of British Columbia in Canada, published a phenomenal body of research on maternity care and place of birth. Some of Kentucky's stats that have come out of that study, compared to national averages, include[20]:

- 35.1% of Kentucky mothers deliver by C-section, while the national average is 32.2%
- 28.1% of Kentucky mothers are induced vs. 23.2%
- 10.7% of Kentucky babies are born prematurely vs. 9.6%
- 8.8% of Kentucky babies are of low birth weight vs. 8.0%
- 42.6 of Kentucky mothers experience spontaneous vaginal birth vs. 49.2%
- 8.6% of Kentucky mothers have a VBAC vs. 11.3%

- 66.7% of Kentucky mothers are breastfeeding at birth vs. 80.3%
- 16.8% of Kentucky mothers are breastfeeding at six months vs. 24.9%

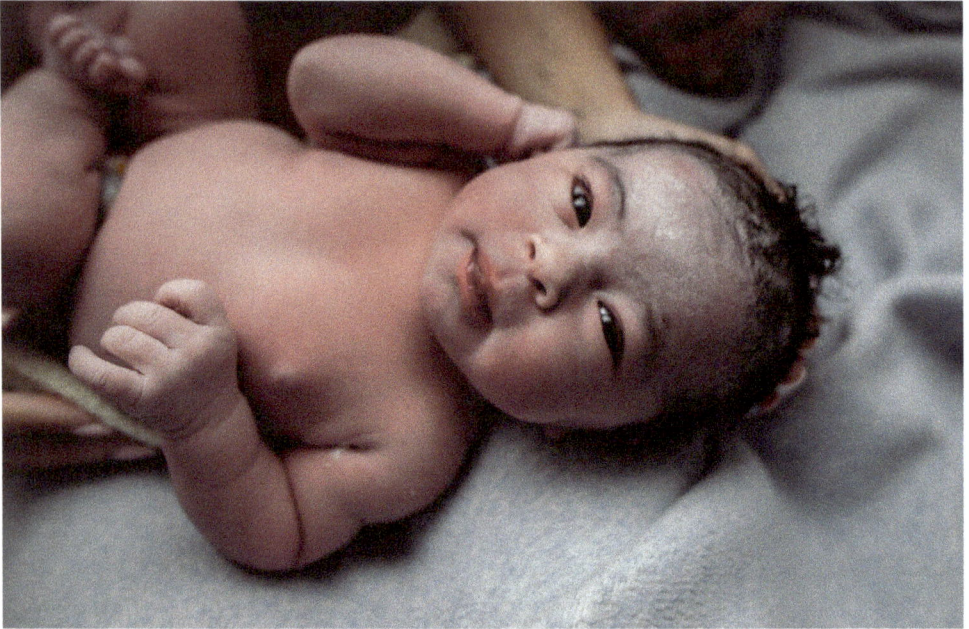

Copyright © 2019 Katie Lacer/MommaKTShoots

Overall, Kentucky's 2018 maternal mortality average is 19.4 deaths per 100,000 live births, while the U.S. average is 20.7.[21] That average is 42.1 deaths for Kentucky's black women compared to 17.2 deaths for white women – even as black women make up less than 5% of Kentucky's population[22]. We must take serious heed to these outcomes. Healthy moms and healthy babies create healthy communities.

Section II: Other Dilemmas: Money, Hospital Closures, the Need in Rural Areas, and Medicaid

Against this backdrop, the U.S. remains the most expensive place on the planet to give birth. For example, our average total hospital and physician costs for a normal delivery is 270% more than in the United Kingdom and 332% more than Spain.[23] For a C-Section, those figures are 239% and 386%, respectively.

The standard two-day hospital stay after delivery accounts for 83% of the total costs associated with a birth. That means the nine months leading up to the birth and out-of-hospital postpartum care only is only responsible for 17 cents of each dollar spent for a pregnancy.[24]

American hospitals charge patients with employer-provided insurance about $32,000 on average for natural births and $51,000 for Cesarean sections. What is the actual estimated amount that insurers agree to pay providers? For vaginal delivery, the prices ranged from $5,017 in Alabama to $10,413 in Alaska.[25] For C-sections, the prices ranged from $7,439 in Washington, DC to $14,528 in Alaska.

In Kentucky, that figure is $5,905 for vaginal delivery and $8,773 for Cesarean.

In contrast, a home birth in Kentucky can range anywhere from $2,000 to $7,000, depending on the midwife, what area she is located in, and her experience.[26] Midwife-attended births at home and in birth centers cost approximately one-third less than hospital deliveries, the latter of which account for $86 billion a year of U.S. healthcare costs.[27]

Another dilemma is the fact that hospitals are shutting down, leaving fewer options for mothers. Of America's 1,984 rural counties, representing 18 million women of reproductive age living in those areas, 45% of them had no hospitals with obstetric services in 2004.[28] By 2014, that figure had jumped to 54%.

In Kentucky, about 41% of the population lives in a rural area.[29] This creates more restricted access to not only critical hospitals, but also to clinics that can adequately support expectant mothers and babies.

Money plays a key role, including the cost to have a bed, equipment, and skilled staff ready 24/7 for a baby to be born. When rural hospitals close the doors of their maternity units, women have to drive longer distances to access care. As if that wasn't enough, in 2015 three hospitals banded together to ensure that no birth center would operate in Kentucky. Mary Carol Akers, a CPM, spent over a quarter of a million dollars attempting to get this birth center for women.[30] In the end, it got shut it down through the appeals process in court, by hospitals who could outspend her in their legal efforts.

Despite declines in hospital-based obstetric services in many rural communities, midwifery care at home and in free-standing birth centers can be and is an available option. Rural areas have higher rates of chronic conditions that make pregnancy more challenging, higher rates of childbirth-related hemorrhages, and higher rates of maternal and infant deaths.[31] Midwives can help address and reverse all of these outcomes in an environment with fewer resources.

In fact, one study examined maternal and neonatal outcomes among planned home and birth center births attended by midwives, comparing outcomes for rural and nonrural women.[32] With a total of 18,723 low-risk, planned home and birth center births, outcomes of 3,737 rural women were compared to outcomes of nonrural women. Maternal outcomes

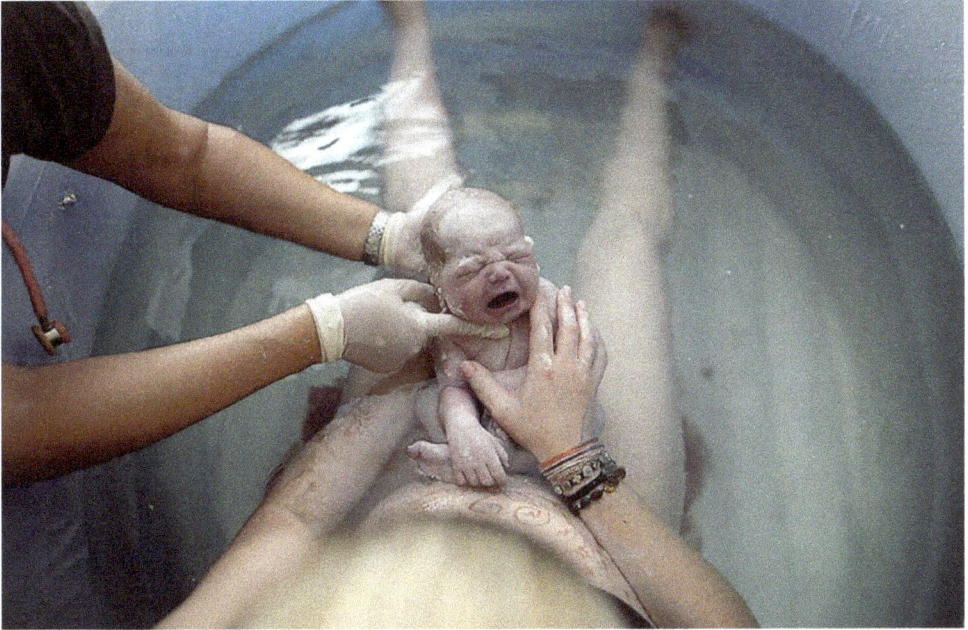

Copyright © 2019 Katie Lacer/MommaKTShoots

included mode of delivery (Cesarean and instrumental delivery), blood transfusions, severe events, perineal lacerations, transfer to hospital, and a composite (any of the above). The conclusion? "Among this sample of low-risk women who planned midwife-led community births, no increased risk was detected by rural vs nonrural status."

It's also worthy to note that because rural counties tend to be poorer, any efforts to revamp or slash Medicaid could hit mothers especially hard. Medicaid funds almost half of all births in the nation,[33] and the largest increases in Medicaid as the source of payment for deliveries is for women aged 30 and over.[34]

About 44% of all Kentucky births were paid for by Medicaid in 2010.[35] State and federal programs to support the rural maternity workforce are crucial.

These programs should support training in emergency births in rural communities that lose obstetric care, and support the costs of providing maternity care in communities where there are willing providers.

Currently, services rendered by Certified Professional Midwives (CPMs) are not recognized under Medicaid at the federal level. However, 13 states have opted, through a state plan amendment, to cover CPM services.[36] A study using data from Washington state's Department of Social and Health Services found that, on average, a home birth attended by a CPM cost Medicaid $2,171 less than a low-risk hospital birth.[37] That was as of 2004. In 2019 dollars, that would be $2,951.[38]

The study sought to determine whether the costs of administering the state's midwife licensing program are offset by economic benefits of the care provided by CPMs. Figures incorporated all costs associated with CPM care, including those associated with hospital transfers when necessary. The total savings of the practice of licensed midwifery on the cost of deliveries to all taxpayers was estimated to be $1.36 million per year, which is almost 10 times the cost to license CPMs. This is the total cost savings to Washington's healthcare system (public and private insurance).

The Midwives and Mothers in Action (MAMA) Campaign and the American College of Nurse-Midwives (ACNM) have both called for Medicaid payment/reimbursement for midwifery services, with the ACNM stating specifically, "Reimbursement from third party payers should be available to licensed maternity care providers for home birth services."[39] [40]

And for physicians and hospitals concerned about rising malpractice insurance rates if midwives are allowed to freely practice and integrate within the healthcare system, this may not be as much of a concern as posed.

Ann Geisler runs Southern Cross Insurance Solutions, which specializes in insuring midwives. She says her clients' premiums tend to be just one-tenth of premiums for an OB-GYN because their model of care eschews unnecessary interventions or technology.[41] "Generally, licensed midwives only treat low-risk women… If the patients become higher risk, midwives are supposed to transfer them to a doctor's care," says Geisler.

Section III: What We Can Learn From the 'Gold Standard'

Some researchers, like Dr. William Callaghan, chief of the Maternal and Infant Health Branch of the Centers for Disease Control and Prevention (CDC), describe the U.K. as having the "gold standard for maternal health data."[42]

There, health care practitioners review every maternal death, using medical records and more to identify deaths related to pregnancy or childbirth as well as to determine why they happened and if better care could have prevented them. Not only are review committees put in place, but standard procedures in the event of a life-threatening incident are as well.

Kate Womersley detailed this in her co-published article with NPR for ProPublica titled, "Why giving birth is safer in Britain than in the U.S."[43] She shared the story of Helen Taylor, who gave birth to twins by Cesarean in June 2017 in England. In the midst of complications where Helen lost over a third of her blood, her team – an obstetrician and her resident in training, a pediatrician, an anesthesiologist with an assistant, two nurses, and three midwives (about half of all babies born in Great Britain are delivered by midwife) – responded with precision by following standard procedures.

British doctors must follow the same guidelines for many aspects of maternity care, like postpartum hemorrhage guidelines that are regularly updated by the Royal College of Obstetricians and Gynecologists and The National Institute for Health and Care Excellence. Those guidelines are then written into local protocols for practice in every National Health Service hospital (by the way, virtually the entire population is covered under the National Health Service and services are free, financed primarily through general taxes, except for certain minor charges).[44] You don't need to be a doctor to read the guidelines; they are freely available online at www.rcog.org.uk/guidelines.

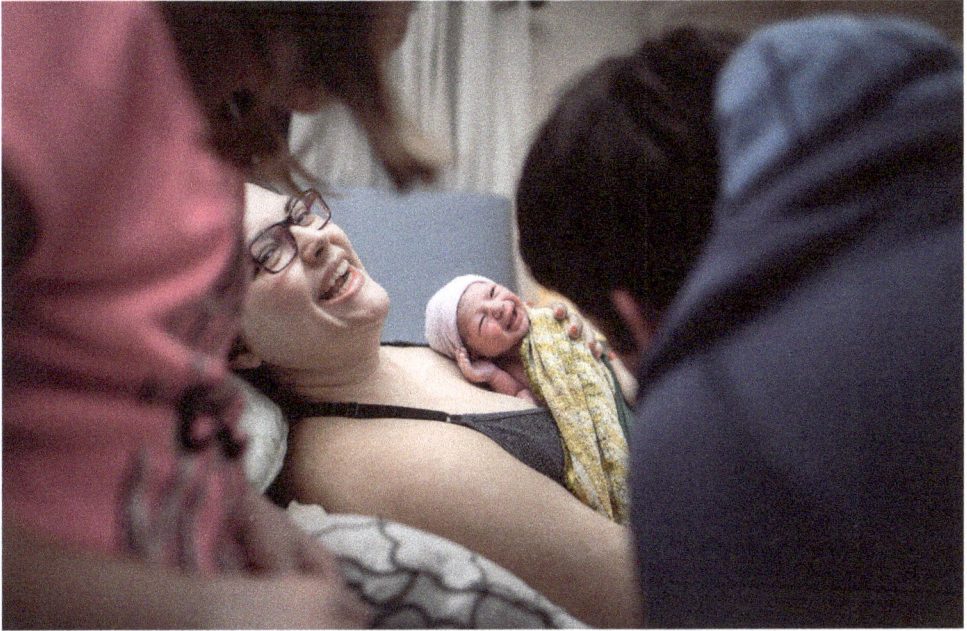

Copyright © 2018 Katie Lacer/MommaKTShoots

On December 11, 2018, we took a step in the right direction when the U.S. House of Representatives passed H.R.1318 "Preventing Maternal Deaths Act of 2018," and then the Senate did the same two days later[45]. The bill was promoted heavily by Charles Johnson IV, who lost his wife Kira in 2016 hours after she had delivered their second child by C-section in a terrible case of negligence.[46]

H.R. 1318 will be our national law requiring review of maternal deaths. All 50 states will receive funding (a total of $60 million over five years) to:

- Establish maternal mortality review committees that collect information and investigate maternal deaths;
- Implement plans and recommendations for ongoing health care provider education to improve outcomes; and
- Provide public disclosure of information included in state reports, including allowing for voluntary reporting of such deaths by family members

The Alliance for Innovation on Maternal Health (AIM) gives physicians a head start on what may be coming from this new bill. AIM formalized safety practices shown to reduce maternal injuries into a series of "safety bundles" that detail treatment policies, safety equipment, training programs and internal reviews every maternity hospital should have like setting time deadlines for taking blood pressure readings and administering medications to pregnant women and new moms experiencing dangerously high blood pressure.[47]

The bundles have been sponsored by a coalition of leading medical societies whose members include American College of Obstetricians and Gynecologists (ACOG), the ACNM, and the American Academy of Family Physicians (AAFP).

One Major Difference

As the story above of Helen Taylor highlights, one key difference in the medical system in the U.K. versus the U.S. is the integration of midwives. Thought of as a thing of the past here in the States, midwives are very much utilized in other developed nations. In Sweden, Norway, and France, for example, midwives oversee most expectant and new mothers, enabling obstetricians to concentrate on high-risk births. In Canada and New Zealand, midwives are so highly valued that they're brought in to manage complex cases that need special attention.[48]

These developed nations do not see birth as a medical emergency or event.[49] Rather, birth is seen as a physiologic event – a natural, everyday occurrence. As such, the delivery approach is entered into drastically different than in the U.S., including the widespread use of midwives.

While midwives attend 9.9 percent of births in the U.S.[50] (whether in the hospital, birth clinic, or at home; and whether by certified nurse-midwife or certified professional midwife), all planned births in the U.K., from home deliveries to complex C-sections, are attended by midwives. The NHS employs over 21,000 midwives, compared with 4,710 OB-GYNs. Unlike obstetric nurses in the U.S., midwives in Britain do not work under the auspices of obstetricians. Midwives are independent practitioners in their own right, but trained to recognize when a woman or her baby is in trouble and needs an obstetrician's support.

So let's jump into this talk of midwives…

Section IV: A Look at Midwives, Including Certified Professional Midwives

Almost all Americans were born at home in 1900,[51] delivered by midwives. Midwives were valued members of their communities until the late 19th century, when medicine became professionalized and doctors' groups began pushing for a monopoly over obstetric care. With technological advancements, big business backed hospitals and made a concerted effort to move birth from the home with midwives to the hospital with obstetricians. Fierce marketing campaigns painted these midwives as uneducated, unsafe, and too dirty to attend births.

Midwifery began to make a comeback in the 1970s and 80s, on the heels of the feminist movement and the hippie era. It was embraced by middle-class white women who wanted more of a voice in their maternity care and who challenged the status quo to take charge over their own bodies. Today, it remains largely married, college-educated white women who are choosing provider care with midwives in the home birth setting.[52] Many of them also pay for midwifery services out-of-pocket (for a number of reasons), and they are electing home birth after having given birth previously.[53]

Who are midwives?
The Midwives Alliance of North America (MANA), our continent's professional midwifery association, defines midwives as "trained professionals with expertise and skills in supporting women to maintain healthy pregnancies and have optimal births and recoveries during the postpartum period."[54] Furthermore, midwifery is "a woman-centered empowering

model of maternity care that has at its core the characteristics of being with women, listening to women, and sharing knowledge and decision-making with women." That includes four key tenets[55]:

- Monitoring the physical, psychological and social well-being of the mother throughout the childbearing cycle;
- Providing the mother with individualized education, counseling, and prenatal care, continuous hands-on assistance during labor and delivery, and postpartum support;
- Minimizing technological interventions; and
- Identifying and referring women who require obstetrical attention

MANA states that 80% of people alive today have been born with midwives, and in many industrialized nations around the world, midwives

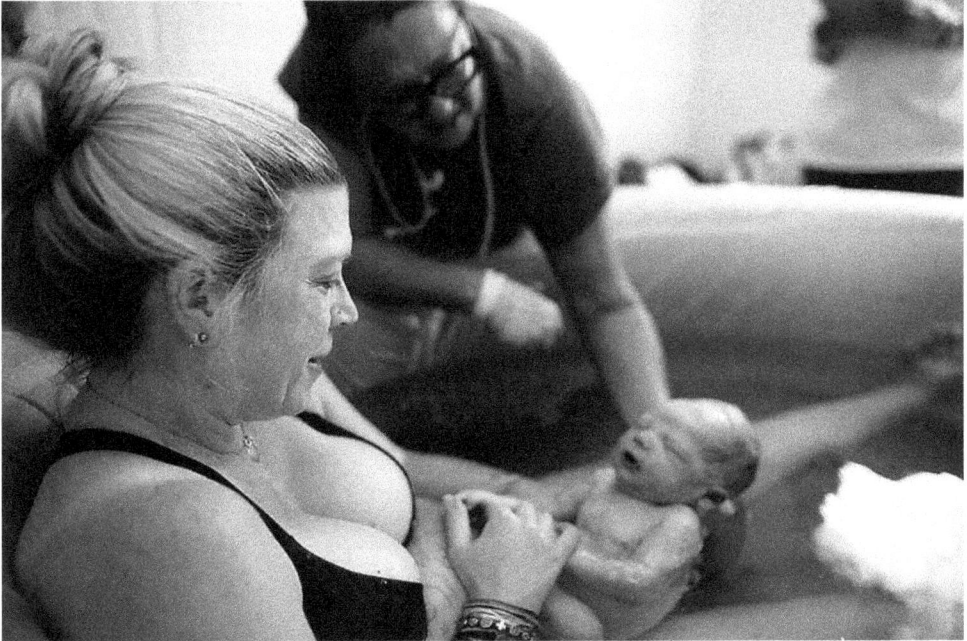

Copyright © 2019 Katie Lacer/MommaKTShoots

attend approximately 70% of all births.[56] "The countries with the lowest mortality and morbidity rates for mothers and infants are those in which midwifery is a valued and integral pillar of the maternity care system," the organization writes. "The midwifery model is a low-tech, high-caring model that produces excellent outcomes not only for low risk women, but for vulnerable and at-risk women as well."

The result of midwifery care on American births?[57] Well, take your pick:

- Lower cost
- Savings to Medicaid
- Lower C-section rates
- Lower rates of induction and augmentation
- Significant reduction in the incidence of third- and fourth-degree perineal tears
- Higher rates of breastfeeding
- Fewer technological interventions
- Significantly higher chance for a normal vaginal birth
- Lower rates of episiotomy
- Fewer pre-term babies
- Fewer low birth weight babies
- Increased access to care, particularly for women of rural areas or underserved/underprivileged communities
- High levels of satisfaction for the mother
- An increased sense of control during the labor and birth experience

The care of midwives is uniquely nurturing, providing women with individualized care suited to their physical, mental, emotional, spiritual and cultural needs. They promote both informed consent and informed refusal in healthcare decision making. They are also trained to detect "yellow flags" and refer women to an obstetrician when needed.

Midwives work in all settings (homes, clinics, freestanding birth centers, and hospitals). In different states, different types of midwives are licensed to practice. Here in Kentucky, we primarily see certified nurse-midwives (CNM) and certified professional midwives (CPM). Both credentials are accredited by the National Commission for Certifying Agencies (NCCA).

CNMs and CPMs: Education, Training, and Credentials

By trade, CNMs are registered nurses who go on to earn a graduate degree, typically catered towards midwifery. They work in all birth settings – hospitals, homes, birth centers and offices – with the majority being in the hospital.

CNMs offer full range of primary health care services for women from adolescence beyond menopause such as: pre-conception care; care during pregnancy, childbirth and the postpartum period; care of the normal newborn during the first 28 days of life; primary care; gynecologic and family planning services; and treatment of male partners for sexually transmitted infections. They also: prescribe medications including controlled substances and contraceptive methods; admit, manage, and discharge patients; order and interpret laboratory and diagnostic tests; and order the use of medical devices.

CNMs showcase their knowledge and skills in accordance with the ACNM's Core Competencies for Basic Midwifery Education.[58] They receive clinical training under the supervision of an American Midwifery Certification Board (AMCB) CNM, Certified Midwife (CM), or other qualified preceptor. They are certified through the Accreditation Commission for Midwifery Education (ACME), under the authorization of the U.S. Department of Education.

CPMs, in contrast, hold the only national midwifery credential that requires knowledge about and experience in out-of-hospital settings, namely homes and freestanding birth centers. In some states, CPMs may also prac-

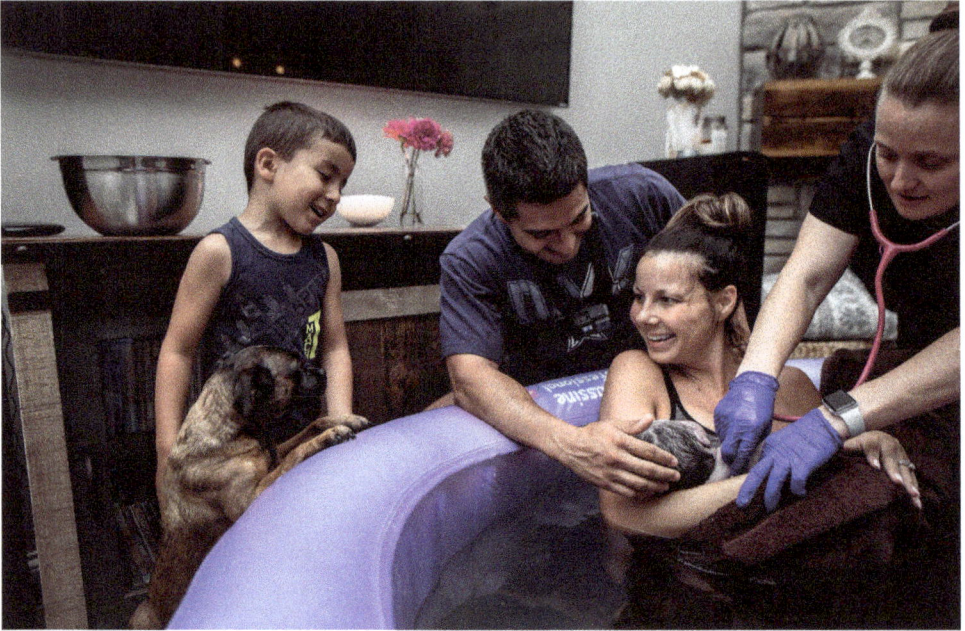

Copyright © 2019 Katie Lacer/MommaKTShoots

tice in clinics and doctors' offices providing well-woman and maternity care. In general, their scope of practice includes care for women in pregnancy, childbirth and the postpartum period, and care of the newborn.

CPMs provide care to women of low-risk profiles who do not have health conditions that should be managed in a hospital. They are trained to recognize abnormal or dangerous conditions requiring consultation with and/ or referral to other health care professionals. They also: conduct physical examinations; administer medications and use devices as allowed by state law; and order and interpret laboratory and diagnostic tests.

CPMs also carry a relatively low client load, averaging three to six births per month, which allows for more personalized and comprehensive care than typical obstetrical practices. For example, prenatal appointments tend to last for an hour or more.

CPMs are certified through the North American Registry of Midwives (NARM), having met the requirements for training, education, and supervised clinical experience, followed by successful completion of a written examination.[59] They complete the pathway for certification either through: a college-granting certificate or degree in midwifery through a Midwifery Education Accreditation Council (MEAC)-accredited school, which is authorized by the U.S. Department of Education; or gaining extensive field experience with a current CPM through the NARM Portfolio Evaluation Process (PEP).

Both pathways for the CPM credential include: attending a minimum of 45 births in a midwifery capacity; conducting a minimum of 100 prenatal exams, 40 newborn exams, and 50 postpartum exams; and completing general coursework on topics like mental health counseling and cultural bias.[60] Apprenticeship includes didactic and clinical training and typically lasts three to five years.

Both pathways also ensure the candidate has met the International Confederation of Midwives (ICM) standards for minimum education for certification. The ICM is the voice of midwives globally. It is a consortium of 500,000 midwives across six continents, including CNMs and CPMs.

While midwives work in all settings, many midwives enjoy the opportunity to deliver babies in the home birth setting…

Section V: The Growing Home Birth Movement

Nationwide, home births have grown – that is, women who plan to birth their children at home instead of at a hospital or a birthing center. As barbaric and archaic as this may sound to someone being presented with this idea for the first time, it is important to note that this trend *is growing*.

Although almost all Americans were born at home in 1900, out-of-hospital births, which largely includes home births, dropped to 44% by 1940 and to 1% by 1969, where it remained until the 1980s. At that point, home births started to creep its way back into American culture, where it has been steadily increasing. Here's a snapshot of recent years:

- Home births grew from 0.56% of all U.S. births in 2004 to 0.72% in 2009[61]

- By 2012, that percentage had jumped to 0.89% home births.[62] The total out-of-hospital births (includes freestanding birthing center, clinic or doctor's office, residence, and other) was 1.36%, its highest level since 1975. Of those 53,635 births in 2012 that occurred out of a hospital, 35,184 were home births and 15,577 were birthing center births.

- By 2016, the home birth percentage was 0.98%[63]

From 2004-2017, home births in the U.S. increased by 77%. Meanwhile, hospital births from that same period decreased by 0.7%.[64] Looking at 2017 specifically, the 0.99% home birth rate represented 38,343 of 3,855,500 total births. The states with the highest home birth rates were Montana at 2.7%, Idaho at 2.3%, Vermont at 2.6%, and Wyoming at 2.3%.[65]

Kentucky's current home birth rate is also above the national average, at 1.35%. Alabama, Nebraska, and Louisiana have the lowest rates, all at 0.3%.

The CDC also notes: "There is evidence that the number of live births attended by certified nurse midwives is understated, largely due to difficulty in correctly identifying the birth attendant when more than one provider is present at the birth. (Anecdotal evidence suggests that some hospitals require that a physician be reported as the attendant even where no physician is physically present at midwife-attended births.)."[66]

So even for the percentages we have of place of birth and birth attendant (i.e. certified nurse-midwife, M.D., other midwife), the percentages may actually be higher for midwife-attended births, including those births that were attended by a CPM but then a transfer to the hospital took place and the birth certificates documents the MD/OB who actually delivered the baby as the "birth attendant".

Kentucky mothers have increasingly opted to give birth at home, in the care of midwives. In 1988, there were 51,422 total births.[67] Of those, 177 were home births (0.34%). In 2016, of Kentucky's 54,662 total births, 738 occurred at home (1.35%). In fact, from 2010 to 2016 alone, home births in Kentucky grew by 38.7%. In contrast, hospital births of that same time period decreased by 2.3%.

Think about that.

What for decades has seemed to be the "normal" standard for birth has not only hovered around stagnant, but has actually decreased. Meanwhile, home births have grown by a third – in just six years.

Since 1988, a total of 11,286 births in Kentucky have occurred at home, most under the care of midwives.

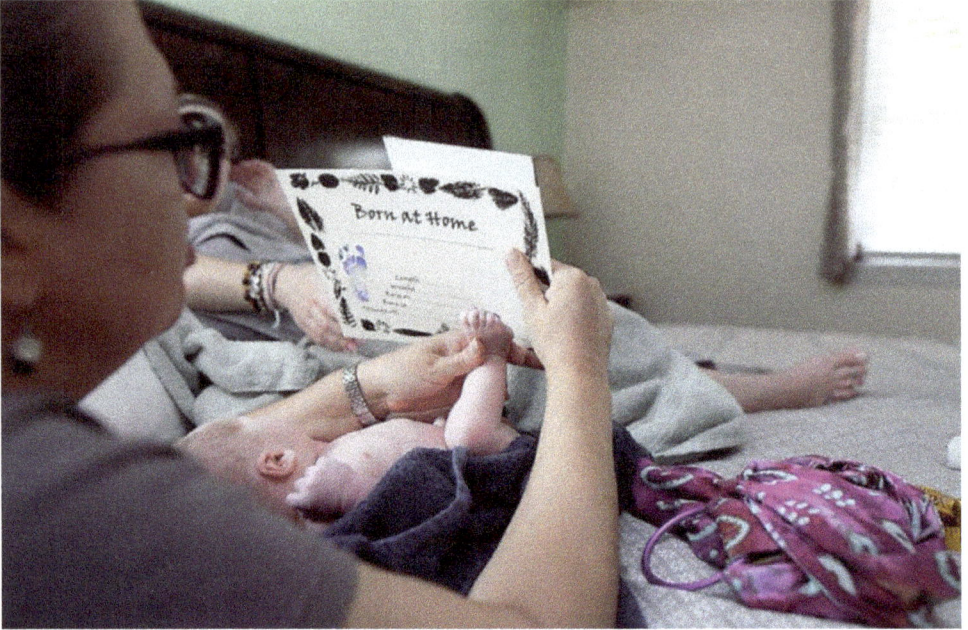

Copyright © 2019 Katie Lacer/MommaKTShoots

Why Home Birth?

Home birth has been shown to contribute to comfort, mobility, ability to cope, and sense of confidence for the mother.[68] Many women actually believe it is safer to give birth at home than at a hospital, where they will avoid unnecessary medical interventions.[69] Even obstetricians who have individually delivered thousands of births in hospitals have been highlighted for choosing to birth their children at home.

"I had an expert midwife who kept meticulous records of her outcomes," says Jennifer Lang, M.D. and board-certified obstetrician-gynecologist who opted for a home birth for her second child.[70] "I've never seen an obstetrician at the first prenatal visit hand over their complete list of how many thousands of births they had done, what their overall C-section rate was, how many complications they had, what the complications were. My midwife did that for me and I felt incredibly safe in her hands. Her statistics were far better than any of the OBs I'd ever met, or even my own."

34

MANA highlights the following on home birth:[71]

- Homebirth is an expression of a woman's autonomy and a process in which her autonomy and privacy are assured.

- At home, a laboring woman is free to be guided instinctively to birth her baby in whatever position feels right, in or out of water, as she desires. The heightened senses of the new mother and baby are stimulated by uninterrupted closeness and familiar voices rather than being disrupted by the jarring lights, noises, and separations that so often occur in an institutional setting. Nursing the newborn in the first hours is undisturbed in the homebirth setting.

- Each birth setting carries a particular set of risks and benefits. Each woman must evaluate which set of risks and benefits are most acceptable to her and most in keeping with her belief system and her family's best interests. There is no significant statistical difference in outcome in terms of maternal or perinatal mortality between hospital and out-of-hospital birth.

- Homebirth preserves skills, knowledge, and ways of knowing in relationship to birth and midwifery practice that are uniquely possible in the home setting, where birth unfolds naturally without routine interference and with only judicious use of technology appropriate to that setting.

Is Home Birth Safe? A Look at the Studies

In the peer-reviewed Journal of Midwifery & Women's Health (JMWH), a landmark study by Cheyney, Bovbjerg, et al. confirmed that among low-risk women, planned home births result in low rates of intervention without an increase in risks for mothers and babies.[72] This study is the largest analysis of planned home birth in the U.S. ever published, examining outcomes of 16,924 planned home births in the U.S. between 2004 and 2009.

In that study, only 1% of babies required transfer to the hospital after birth, the majority of which were for failure to progress. The rates of spontaneous vaginal birth and Cesarean were 93.6% and 5.2%, respectively – all better than hospital outcomes. Of the 1,054 women who attempted a vaginal birth after Cesarean, 87% were successful. Only 1.5% had 5-minute Apgar scores below 7 (a measure of the health of a newborn on a scale of 1-10, with 10 being the best). In comparison, for all U.S. births between 2007 and 2010, of which an average 99.0% of births occurred in the hospital in those same years, that same statistic was 1.8%.[73]

Also in the study, the majority of newborns (86%) were exclusively breast-feeding at six weeks. Excluding lethal anomalies, neonatal mortality rates were 0.76 per 1,000, which is less than the 2017 U.S. average of 3.85 per 1,000 live births.[74]

Additionally, 92% of babies were carried to full-term and they weighed an average of eight pounds at birth. Babies born to low-risk mothers had no higher risk of death in labor or the first few weeks of life than those in comparable studies of similarly low-risk pregnancies.

Another study was conducted in 2000 in North America, including the United States and Canada. In it, 5,418 women supported by midwives with a common certification planned to deliver at home when labor began. Of them, 12.1% were transferred to a hospital.[75] Medical intervention rates included epidural (4.7%), episiotomy (2.1%), forceps (1.0%), vacuum extraction (0.6%), and Cesarean section (3.7%) – all lower than for low-risk U.S. women having hospital births.

Neonatal deaths, excluding those concerning life-threatening congenital anomalies, was 1.7 per 1,000 planned home births, similar to risks in other studies of low-risk home and hospital births in North America. No mothers died. The final conclusion: "Planned home birth for low-risk women in

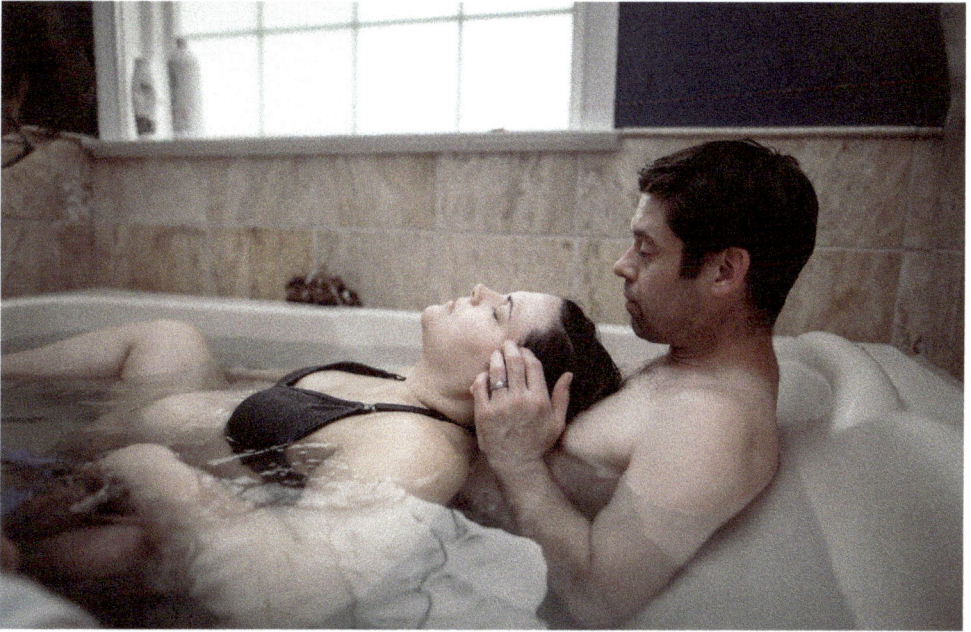

North America using certified professional midwives was associated with lower rates of medical intervention, but similar intrapartum and neonatal mortality to that of low-risk hospital births in the U.S."

In 2001, the Birthplace in England Collaborative Group reported findings from a study of 64,538 births among low-risk women in England. Investigators concluded that for healthy women, adverse maternal and newborn outcomes were extremely rare, regardless of birth setting.[76]

In 2008, a meta-analysis on the safety of home birth in the western world took a look at six controlled observational studies that included a total of 24,092 primarily low-risk pregnant women.[77] The principal difference in the outcome was a lower frequency of low Apgar scores and severe lacerations in the home birth group. Fewer medical interventions occurred in the home birth group including induction, augmentation, episiotomy, and

Cesarean section. No maternal deaths occurred in the studies. The conclusion: "Home birth is an acceptable alternative to hospital confinement for selected pregnant women, and leads to reduced medical interventions."

A study of all planned home births attended by midwives in British Columbia, Canada from 2000 to 2004 revealed no increase in neonatal mortality over planned hospital births attended by either midwives or physicians.[78] Interesting note: Registered midwives in British Columbia are mandated to offer women the choice to deliver in a hospital or at home if they meet the eligibility criteria for home birth defined by the College of Midwifery of British Columbia.

Over in Ontario, Canada, another study evaluated the difference in outcomes between planned home and planned hospital births. The researchers used a provincial database of all midwifery-booked pregnancies between 2006 and 2009 to compare women who planned home birth at the onset of labor to a matched cohort of women with low-risk pregnancies who had planned hospital births attended by midwives. They compared 11,493 planned home births and 11,493 planned hospital births.[79] The result? All intrapartum interventions were lower among planned home births. "Compared with planned hospital birth, planned home birth attended by midwives in a jurisdiction where home birth is well-integrated into the health care system was not associated with a difference in serious adverse neonatal outcomes, but was associated with fewer intrapartum interventions."

And a 2014 nationwide cohort study from the Netherlands compared outcomes of 466,112 women who had a planned home birth and 276,958 who had a planned hospital birth.[80] The conclusion? "We found no increased risk of adverse perinatal outcomes for planned home births among low-risk women. Our results may only apply to regions where home births are well integrated into the maternity care system."

So, the studies we have show that home birth with certified midwives is not dangerous, especially if the planned home birth and midwives are well-integrated into the larger healthcare system. Studies show, in fact, that home birth often leads to healthier outcomes than hospitals.

Home Birth Position Statements

Home birth has become so popular and has grown as a viable option that ACOG and the American Academy of Pediatrics (AAP) have weighed in on it. ACOG's Committee Opinion dated April 2017 states some of the following excerpts:[81]

"Although the American College of Obstetricians and Gynecologists believes that hospitals and accredited birth centers are the safest settings for birth, each woman has the right to make a medically informed decision about delivery."

This excerpt is important to note because this opinion replaced ACOG's sharply-worded 2007 policy statement that declared "ACOG does not support programs or individuals that advocate for or who provide home births."[82] Essentially, ACOG shifted from an absolute "no" to "women should have freedom of choice".

Continuing, "Importantly, women should be informed that several factors are critical to reducing perinatal mortality rates and achieving favorable home birth outcomes. These factors include the appropriate selection of candidates for home birth; the availability of a certified nurse–midwife, certified midwife or midwife whose education and licensure meet International Confederation of Midwives' Global Standards for Midwifery Education, or physician practicing obstetrics within an integrated and regulated health system; ready access to consultation; and access to safe and timely transport to nearby hospitals."

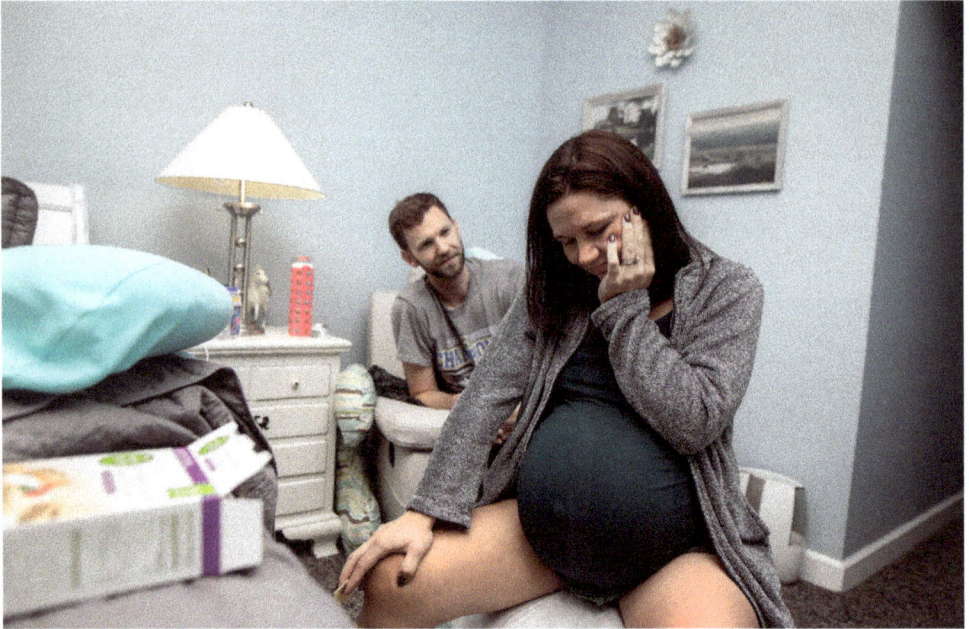

Copyright © 2018 Katie Lacer/MommaKTShoots

AGOC states, "The relative risk versus benefit of a planned home birth, however, remains the subject of debate. High-quality evidence that can inform this debate is limited. To date, there have been no adequate randomized clinical trials of planned home birth." This is ACOG's statement, perhaps alluding to the belief that MANA's study of nearly 17,000 women is not sufficient.

Continuing, "Women inquiring about planned home birth should be informed of its risks and benefits based on recent evidence. Specifically, they should be informed that although planned home birth is associated with fewer maternal interventions than planned hospital birth, it also is associated with a more than twofold increased risk of perinatal death (1–2 in 1,000) and a threefold increased risk of neonatal seizures or serious neurologic dysfunction (0.4–0.6 in 1,000)." In spite of this, ACOG says, "the absolute risks remain low."

ACOG goes on to say, "Recent studies have found that when compared with planned hospital births, planned home births are associated with fewer maternal interventions, including labor induction or augmentation, regional analgesia, electronic fetal heart rate monitoring, episiotomy, operative vaginal delivery, and Cesarean delivery. Planned home births also are associated with fewer vaginal, perineal, and third-degree or fourth-degree lacerations and less maternal infectious morbidity."

ACOG also states, "The College believes that the availability of timely transfer and an existing arrangement with a hospital for such transfers is a requirement for consideration of a home birth. When antepartum, intrapartum, or postpartum transfer of a woman from home to a hospital occurs, the receiving health care provider should maintain a nonjudgmental demeanor with regard to the woman and those individuals accompanying her to the hospital. A characteristic common to those cohort studies reporting comparable rates of perinatal mortality is the provision of care by uniformly highly educated and trained certified midwives who are well integrated into the health care system…"

This is actually a practice that occurs in many areas around the country, like a community in Minneapolis where home birth midwives whose clients transfer to the hospital are welcome into the hospital and are met with the care of a certified nurse midwife and an obstetrician.[83] Home birth midwives bring the prenatal records and are prepared to do a "handoff" to the hospital staff, while still working closely with the staff. This midwife-to-midwife transfer is very appealing to home birth providers and their patients.

In Washington, midwives often collaborate closely with OB-GYNs, and can generally transfer care to hospitals smoothly when risks to the mother or baby emerge. Midwives sit on the state's perinatal advisory committee, are actively involved in shaping health policy, and receive Medicaid reimbursement for home births.[84] [85]

ACOG does note risk factors for planned home birth, including fetal mal-presentation, multiple gestation, and prior Cesarean delivery. It concurs with the opinion of home birth that includes "…the absence of any preex-isting maternal disease; the absence of significant disease arising during the pregnancy; gestational age greater than 36–37 completed weeks and less than 41–42 completed weeks of pregnancy; labor that is spontaneous or induced as an outpatient; and that the patient has not been transferred from another referring hospital."[86]

AAP's stance on planned home birth is similar to that of ACOG's, "…affirm-ing that hospitals and birthing centers are the safest settings for birth in the United States while respecting the right of women to make a medically informed decision about delivery."[87]

It goes on to state, "This statement is intended to help pediatricians pro-vide supportive, informed counsel to women considering home birth while retaining their role as child advocates and to summarize the standards of care for newborn infants born at home, which are consistent with stan-dards for infants born in a medical care facility."

How about the ACNM? The organization also echoes in agreement the positions of ACOG and AAP.[88] Furthermore, its "Midwifery Provision of Home Birth Services" paper states, "The number of women in the United States choosing to give birth at home has risen substantially in the past decade, creating an increased need for understanding of the evidence regarding the provision of midwifery care to women and families consid-ering this option. The safety of home birth has been evaluated in observa-tional studies in several industrialized nations, including the United States. Most studies find that women who are essentially healthy at term with a singleton fetus and give birth at home have positive outcomes and a lower rate of interventions during labor. Although some studies have found

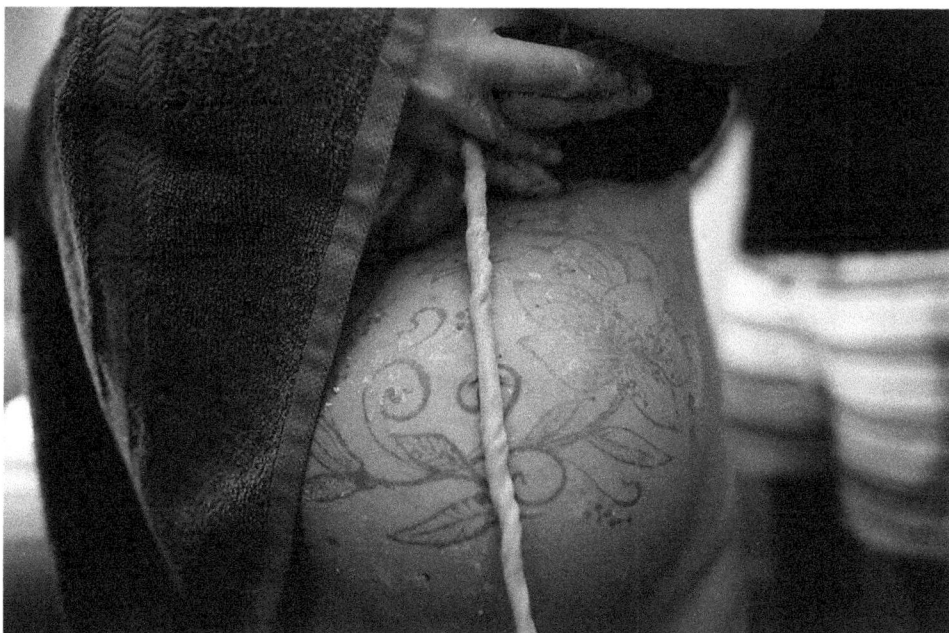

increased neonatal morbidity and mortality in newborns born at home when compared to newborns born in a hospital, the absolute numbers reported in both birth sites are very low."[89]

The conclusion: "International and US research results support the conclusion that planned home birth with an educated, skilled attendant can be a safe, satisfying, cost-effective care option for healthy, low-risk women who want to give birth at home."

Lastly, ICM's position statement on home birth states, "ICM believes that a woman has the right to a home birth as a valid and safe option. ICM underscores the right of women to make an informed decision to give birth at home supported by a midwife. The midwife who provides professional services for women in their homes should be able to do so within a nation's health system and with access to insurance and appropriate compensation. ICM regrets that not all nations have the legislation or health systems

43

which support planned home birth, and urges national governments to review the scientific literature and work towards a maternity care system which includes this option."[90]

Integrating Midwives into the Healthcare System

The Birth Place Lab's five-year study by researchers in the U.S. and Canada shows that states that have done the most to integrate midwives into their health care systems – including Washington, New Mexico and Oregon – have some of the best outcomes for mothers and babies.[91] Conversely, states with some of the most restrictive midwife laws and practices — including Alabama, Ohio and Mississippi — tend to do significantly worse on key indicators of maternal and neonatal well-being.

In Washington, CPMs have a number of benefits including the fact that they are licensed to practice and they have easy access to a physical referral.[92] They are even covered by Medicaid.

In New Mexico, as of 2013, 1.3% of all births occurred at home. CPMs there have the same freedoms as CPMs in Washington. Midwives in general, including CPMs and CNMs, attend 26.4% of all births in New Mexico.[93] It's also worthy to note that New Mexico has the lowest rates of C-section of all 50 states.

In Oregon, 2.5% of all births occur at home – almost double that of Kentucky.[94] Looking at indicators like C-section rate, induction rate, premature births, low birth weight, and neonatal mortality, all of these Oregon statistics fare better than the U.S. average. And for positive indicators like spontaneous vaginal birth, VBAC, breastfeeding at birth, and breastfeeding at six months, Oregon's statistics also fare better than the national average.

What about transfers? A big question around home births is how the transfer from home to hospital will work if needed.

In Washington, for example, a group of physicians and midwives formed The Physician-Midwife Workgroup, a multidisciplinary subcommittee of the Washington State Perinatal Collaborative (WSPC).[95] This workgroup developed a quality improvement project initiative called Smooth Transitions to enhance the safety of planned out-of-hospital birth transports.[96]

That committee is made up of doctors, licensed midwives, nurses, a state department of health representative, a state hospital association representative, a public state university medical center representative, a healthcare consumer, and an EMS representative. The model has improved communications between partners and is adaptable to individual hospitals across the nation.

Section VI: The Legalities of Birth and Midwifery in Kentucky

Over 700 families per year have planned home births in Kentucky, which is a growing trend, even as hospital births have declined. Overwhelmingly, the care providers who attend these home births are CPMs.

Since 1975, CPMs have not been licensed to practice. Kentucky issued permits (as a form of licensure) to midwives from the 1950s until 1975, when the Kentucky Cabinet for Health and Family Services stopped issuing them for reasons unknown.[97] And we were not alone. Up until earlier this year, 18 states still did not license CPMs.

As a result, CPMs in Kentucky have practiced "underground" with immeasurable legal liability and restriction. This legal limitation has also drastically reduced the number of CPMs in Kentucky who attend home births – in an era where home birth is now evidenced to be a safe option for low-risk women. As of late 2018, there were only seven resident CPMs accepting new patients in the entire state of Kentucky, which has about 54,000 total births per year. Fourteen additional CPMs from neighboring states provide home birth care for Kentucky women. This is disheartening, particularly in western Kentucky where there is no CPM available. In Louisville, the most populous city in the state, there is only one practicing resident CPM.

However, the change is here. Led by the Kentucky Home Birth Coalition (KHBC), a strong, grassroots campaign for licensure was created in 2012, including: educating the general public on midwifery care; connecting with legislators; hosting fundraisers; and hosting community meetings across the state.

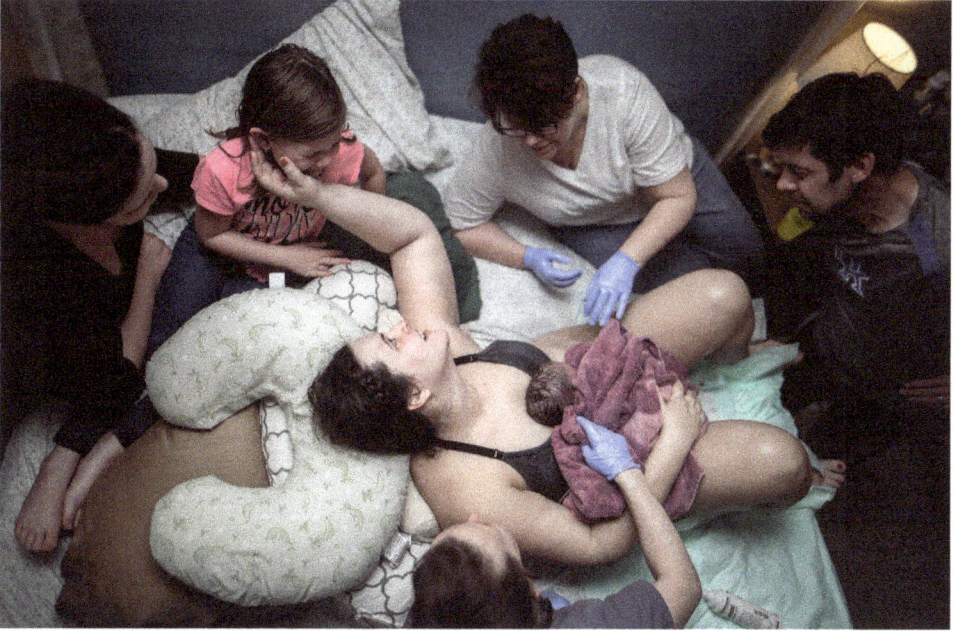
Copyright © 2018 Katie Lacer/MommaKTShoots

Senate Bill (SB) 84, "An Act related to licensed certified professional midwives", sponsored by Senator Buford (R-District 22), is the work of the KHBC. On March 26, 2019, the bill was passed through the Kentucky Senate after having passed out of the House during the General Session.

SB84: An Act Relating to Licensed Certified Professional Midwives

The goal was to have the government of Kentucky begin issuing licenses again. The bipartisan SB 84 passed out of the Senate's Health and Welfare Committee in 2018,[98] [99] but was derailed by a Special Session. It came back up for a vote in the House in February 2019 and passed 96-1. It then received a favorable 35-1 vote to pass out of the Senate in March. It was signed by Governor Matt Bevin on March 26, 2019.

The bill, now enacted into law, will allow for the state issuance of licenses for CPMs, as well as a number of benefits like:[100]

- Create a diverse CPM Advisory Council under the Board of Nursing, including midwives, physicians and Advanced Practice Registered Nurses (APRN), to advise on matters including competency determination, necessary statutory changes, and limitations on practice;

- Allow CPMs to order medical tests necessary to confirm that home birth is a safe option, and establish a specific list of critical safety medications that CPMs may obtain and administer (but not prescribe), such as medication to manage sudden postpartum hemorrhage;

- Integrate CPMs into the existing healthcare system, allowing open communication with other healthcare practitioners such as Obstetricians and Pediatricians;

- Create requirements for home-to-hospital transfers. Midwives will be able to openly identify themselves as caregivers to hospital personnel, medical records can be transferred and accepted, and transfers will happen sooner as families will not be fearful of a hostile hospital environment.

Next Steps

Now that SB 84 has been enacted into law, families planning to have a home birth in Kentucky can soon solicit CPMs who are officially licensed. The stigma of seeking a CPM underground is lifted. The rights, education, and credentials of CPMs are respected. The opportunity for CPMs to be engrained into the larger healthcare system has arrived, including the opportunity for CPMs to bill their home birth clients through insurance instead of those clients having to pay out of pocket for their prenatal care and home birth. This, in turn, makes it easier for women to access midwifery care. Essentially, more Kentuckians are provided the choice and freedom to more readily elect home birth as a viable option.

Section VII: Conclusion: The Voice of the Woman

Women in Kentucky are choosing how and where they give birth. SB84 is a huge step in protecting the rights of those women and the midwives they select. It helps dismantle the unwanted legal ramifications and stigma of choosing to birth at home. The rate of home births is anticipated to only increase from here, as it has been doing for the past 30 years.

Women have been shamed, made fearful, scared into viewing birth as an emergency, as a medical problem. In this society, women have been taught that their bodies are not strong enough to handle birth by themselves, that their bodies were not made for this without emergent medical assistance.

The idea that birth is an emergency requiring medical supervision and intervention has resulted in an expensive maternal health-care system that dedicates millions of dollars to procedures and surgeries that experts describe as unnecessary, while failing to provide accessible care to women who want more autonomy over their pregnant bodies and how they birth.

So, women have and will continue to decide that they will not be silenced. They will not be made fearful. They will not be shamed. They will not be devalued or humiliated. These are their bodies – and they're taking them back.

They're bucking the system. They've traded in their traumatic hospital stories for peace and informed consent at home. They've traded in the long, white hallways with bright fluorescent lighting and constant sounds of monitors for quietness and candles. They traded in ice chip meals for actual food that provides nourishment for lengthy labors.

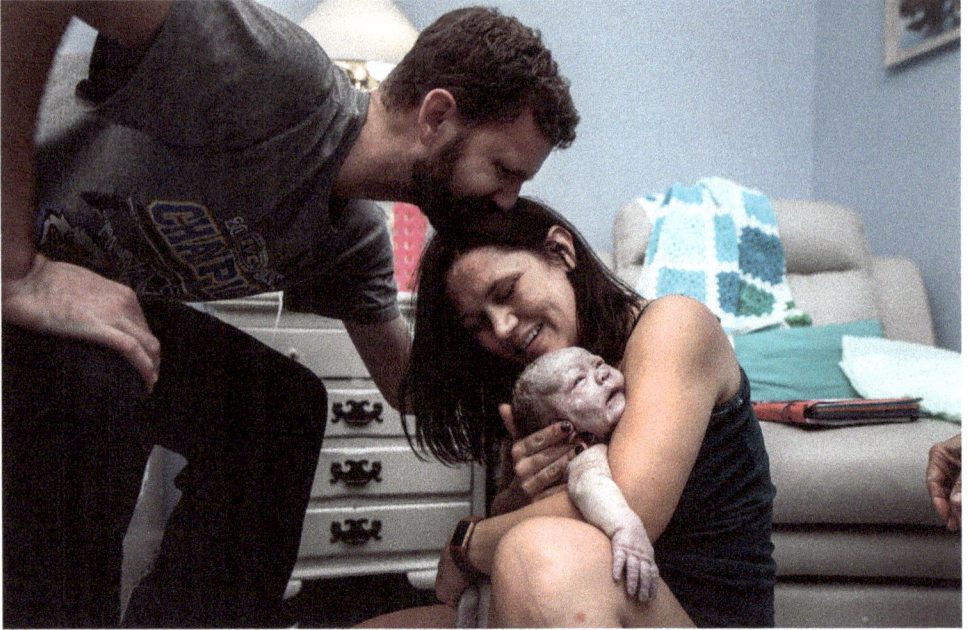

They are enjoying this process that welcomes the beautiful celebration of new life. The growing home birth movement in the state of Kentucky showcases women taking back their power with birth, shifting the birth setting from one that is provider-centered to one that is woman-centered.

Everyone's birth story is different, and every home environment set up to welcome a baby into the world is different. But this is what women are choosing. They are choosing the comfort they find in their homes as the best place to birth – and they have found this to be one of the best decisions of their lives.

Notes

1. Young, A. (2018, July 27). Hospitals know how to protect mothers. They just aren't doing it. *USA Today.* Retrieved from https://www.usatoday.com/ in-depth/news/investigations/deadly-deliveries/2018/07/26/maternal-mortality-rates-preeclampsia-postpartum-hemorrhage-safety/546889002/

2. World Health Organization. (2018, February 16). *Maternal mortality.* Retrieved from http://www.who.int/news-room/fact-sheets/detail/ maternal-mortality

3. World Health Organization. (2018, February 16). *Maternal mortality.* Retrieved from http://www.who.int/news-room/fact-sheets/detail/ maternal-mortality

4. GBD 2015 Maternal Mortality Collaborators. (2015). Global, regional, and national levels of maternal mortality, 1990-2015: A systemic analysis for the Global Burden of Disease Study 2015. *The Lancet.* Retrieved from https:// www.thelancet.com/pdfs/journals/lancet/PIIS0140-6736(16)31470-2.pdf

5. National Center for Health Statistics. (2000). *Report of the panel to evaluate the U.S. standard certificates.* Retrieved from https://www.cdc.gov/nchs/ data/dvs/panelreport_acc.pdf

6. National Vital Statistics Reports. (2016, February 16). Deaths: Final Data for 2013. *Centers for Disease Control and Prevention, 64, 2.* Retrieved from https://www.cdc.gov/nchs/data/nvsr/nvsr64/nvsr64_02.pdf

7. National Vital Statistics Reports. (2011, December 7). Deaths: Final Data for 2008. *Centers for Disease Control and Prevention, 59, 10.* Retrieved from https://www.cdc.gov/nchs/data/nvsr/nvsr59/nvsr59_10.pdf

8. MacDorman, M.F., Declercq, E., Cabral, H., & Morton, C. (2016, September 1). Is the United States maternal mortality rate increasing? Disentangling trends from measurement issues. Obstetrics & Gynecology, 128, 3, 447-455. Retrieved from https://www.ncbi.nlm.nih.gov/pmc/articles/PMC5001799/

9.   Young, A. (2018, July 27). Hospitals know how to protect mothers. They just aren't doing it. *USA Today.* Retrieved from https://www.usatoday.com/ in-depth/news/investigations/deadly-deliveries/2018/07/26/maternal-mortality-rates-preeclampsia-postpartum-hemorrhage-safety/546889002/

10.   Ellison, K., and Martin, N. (2017, December 22). Severe complications for women during childbirth are skyrocketing – and could often be prevented. *ProPublica.* Retrieved from https://www.propublica.org/article/severe-complications-for-women-during-childbirth-are-skyrocketing-and-could-often-be-prevented

11.   Ellison, K., and Martin, N. (2017, December 22). Severe complications for women during childbirth are skyrocketing – and could often be prevented. *ProPublica.* Retrieved from https://www.propublica.org/article/severe-complications-for-women-during-childbirth-are-skyrocketing-and-could-often-be-prevented

12.   Tucker, S. (2018, May 8). There is a hidden epidemic of doctors abusing women in labor, doulas say. *Broadly.* Retrieved from https://broadly.vice.com/en_us/article/evqew7/obstetric-violence-doulas-abuse-giving-birth

13.   American College of Obstetricians and Gynecologists. (2016). *Committee opinion: Refusal of medically recommended treatment during pregnancy.* Retrieved from https://www.acog.org/Clinical-Guidance-and-Publications/Committee-Opinions/Committee-on-Ethics/Refusal-of-Medically-Recommended-Treatment-During-Pregnancy

14.   Lowe, A. (2018, May 11). A doula's call for a 'culture of consent' during childbirth. *WBUR.* Retrieved from http://www.wbur.org/commonhealth/2018/05/11/doula-culture-of-consent

15.   Dekker, R. (2018, February 2). The evidence on: Birthing positions. *Evidence Based Birth.* Retrieved from https://evidencebasedbirth.com/evidence-birthing-positions/

16.   Alfirevic, Z., Devane, D., & Gyte, G. (2006, July 19). Continuous cardiotocography (CTG) as a form of electric fetal monitoring (EFM) for fetal assessment during labour. *PubMed.* doi:10.1002/14651858.CD006066

17.   American Society of Anesthesiologists. (2015, October 25). Most healthy women would benefit from light meal during labor. *ScienceDaily.* Retrieved from https://www.sciencedaily.com/releases/2015/10/151025010725.htm

18.   Dekker, R. (2017). Evidence on: Eating and drinking during labor. *Evidence Based Birth.* Retrieved from https://evidencebasedbirth.com/evidence-eating-drinking-labor/

19.   Ondeck, M. (2014). Health birth practice #2: Walk, move around, and change positions throughout labor. *The Journal of Perinatal Education, 23, 4,* 188-193. doi:10.1891/1058-1243.23.4.188

20.   Birth Place Lab. (2014). Midwifery Integration State Scoring (MISS) system report card: Kentucky. Retrieved from https://www.birthplacelab.org/wp-content/uploads/2018/02/Kentucky.pdf

21.   America's Health Rankings. (2018). Maternal mortality in Kentucky in 2018. *United Health Foundation.* Retrieved from https://www.americashealthrankings.org/explore/health-of-women-and-children/measure/maternal_mortality/state/KY

22.   United States Census Bureau. (2018). *QuickFacts Kentucky.* Retrieved from https://www.census.gov/quickfacts/ky

23.   International Federation of Health Plans. (2012). *2012 Comparative price report: Variation in medical and hospital prices by country.* Retrieved from http://hushp.harvard.edu/sites/default/files/downloadable_files/IFHP%202012%20Comparative%20Price%20Report.pdf

24.   Truven Health Analytics. (2013). *The cost of having a baby in the United States.* Retrieved from http://transform.childbirthconnection.org/wp-content/uploads/2013/01/Cost-of-Having-a-Baby-Executive-Summary.pdf

25.   Rebala, P., & FAIR Health. (2017, October 30). Find out how much it costs to give birth in every state. *Money.* Retrieved from http://money.com/money/4995922/how-much-costs-give-birth-state/

26.   Kentucky Home Birth Coalition. (n.d.). *How much does a home birth cost?* Retrieved from https://kentuckyhomebirthcoalition.com/ufaqs/how-much-does-a-home-birth-cost/

27. National Association of Certified Professional Midwives. (n.d.). *Certified Professional Midwives: Frequently asked questions.* Retrieved from http://nacpm.org/wp-content/uploads/2016/11/CPM_FAQ.pdf

28. Gallardo, A., & Martin, N. (2017, September 5). Another thing disappearing from rural America: Maternal care. *ProPublica.* Retrieved from https://www.propublica.org/article/another-thing-disappearing-from-rural-america-maternal-care

29. Rural Health Information Hub. (2018, January 8). *Kentucky.* Retrieved from https://www.ruralhealthinfo.org/states/kentucky

30. Pascucci, C. (2015, February 26). Kentucky birth monopoly: Begging for birth centers. *Birth Monopoly.* Retrieved from http://birthmonopoly.com/kentuckybirthcenters/

31. Maron, D.F. (2017, February 15). Maternal health care is disappearing in rural America. *Scientific American.* Retrieved from https://www.scientificamerican.com/article/maternal-health-care-is-disappearing-in-rural-america/

32. Nethery, E., Gordon, W., Bovbjerg, M., & Cheyney, M. (2017, November 13). Rural community birth: Maternal and neonatal outcomes for planned community births among rural women in the United States, 2004-2009. Birth: Issues in Perinatal Care, 45, 2, 120-129. https://doi.org/10.1111/birt.12322

33. National Vital Statistics Reports. (2018, January 31). Births: Final Data for 2016. *Centers for Disease Control and Prevention, 67, 1.* Retrieved from https://www.cdc.gov/nchs/data/nvsr/nvsr67/nvsr67_01.pdf

34. Martin, J., Hamilton, B., & Osterman, M. (2018). Births in the United States, 2017. *Centers for Disease Control and Prevention.* Retrieved from https://www.cdc.gov/nchs/data/databriefs/db318.pdf

35. National Vital Statistics Reports. (2013, December 19). Source of payment for the delivery: Births in a 33-state and District of Columbia reporting area, 2010. *Centers for Disease Control and Prevention, 62, 5.* Retrieved from https://www.cdc.gov/nchs/data/nvsr/nvsr62/nvsr62_05.pdf

36. National Association of Certified Professional Midwives. (2016). *Certified professional midwives: Frequently asked questions.* Retrieved from http://nacpm.org/wp-content/uploads/2016/11/CPM_FAQ.pdf

37. Health Management Associates. (2007, October 31). *Midwifery licensure and discipline program in Washington state: Economic costs and benefits.* Retrieved from https://www.washingtonmidwives.org/uploads/1/1/3/8/113879963/midwifery_cost_study_10-31-07.pdf

38. U.S. Inflation Calculator. (2018). Retrieved from https://www.usinflationcalculator.com/

39. Midwives and Mothers in Action Campaign. (n.d.). Reform Medicaid to reduce costs and improve maternity care quality by giving patients choice of providers. *National Association of Certified Professional Midwives (NACPM).* Retrieved from http://nacpm.org/documents/CPMs%20&%20Medicaid%20Reform.pdf

40. American College of Nurse-Midwives. (2011). *Position statement: Home birth.* Retrieved from http://www.midwife.org/ACNM/files/ACNMLibraryData/UPLOADFILENAME/000000000251/Home%20Birth%20Aug%202011.pdf

41. Martin, N. (2018, February 22). A larger role for midwives could improve deficient U.S. care for mothers and babies. *ProPublica.* Retrieved from https://www.propublica.org/article/midwives-study-maternal-neonatal-care

42. Fields, R., & Sexton, J. (2017, October 23). How many American women die from causes related to pregnancy and childbirth? No one knows. *ProPublica.* Retrieved from https://www.propublica.org/article/how-many-american-women-die-from-causes-related-to-pregnancy-or-childbirth

43. Womersley, K. (2017, August 31). Why giving birth is safe in the Britain than in the U.S. *ProPublica.* Retrieved from https://www.propublica.org/article/why-giving-birth-is-safer-in-britain-than-in-the-u-s

44. Britannica. (n.d.). *National Health Service.* Retrieved from https://www.britannica.com/topic/National-Health-Service

45. 115th Congress. (2018). H.R. 1318 Preventing Maternal Deaths Act of 2018. *United States House of Representatives*. Retrieved from https://www. congress.gov/bill/115th-congress/house-bill/1318

46. Chuck, E. (2018, December 19). 'An amazing first step': Advocates hail Congress's maternal mortality prevention bill. *NBC News*. Retrieved from https://www.nbcnews.com/news/us-news/amazing-first-step-advocates-hail-congress-s-maternal-mortality-prevention-n948951

47. Alliance for Innovation on Maternal Health. (2019). What is AIM? *Alliance for Innovation on Maternal Health*. Retrieved from https://safehealthcare-foreverywoman.org/aim-program/

48. Martin, N. (2018, February 22). A larger role for midwives could improve deficient U.S. care for mothers and babies. *ProPublica*. Retrieved from https://www.propublica.org/article/midwives-study-maternal-neonatal-care

49. Santa Cruz, J. (2015, June 12). Call the midwife: Why a growing number of U.S. mothers are turning to midwives, rather than physicians, for prenatal care, labor, and delivery. *The Atlantic*. Retrieved from https://www.theatlantic.com/health/archive/2015/06/midwives-are-making-a-comeback/395456/

50. Centers for Disease Control and Prevention. (2018, November 7). Births: Final data for 2017. Retrieved from https://www.cdc.gov/nchs/data/nvsr/nvsr67/nvsr67_08_tables-508.pdf

51. MacDorman, M., Mathews, T.J., & Declercq, E. (2014). Trends in out-of-hospital births in the United States, 1990-2012. *Centers for Disease Control and Prevention*. Retrieved from https://www.cdc.gov/nchs/products/databriefs/db144.htm

52. Descieux, K., Kavasseri, K., Scott, K., & Parlier, A.B. (2017). Why women choose home birth: A narrative review. *MAHEC Online Journal of Research, 3, 2*. Retrieved from https://sys.mahec.net/media/onlinejournal/why_women.pdf

53. Cheyney, M., Bovbjerg, M., Everson, C., Gordon, W., Hannibal, D., & Vedam, S. (2014, January 30). Outcomes of care for 16,924 planned home births in

the United States: The Midwives Alliance of North America Statistics Project, 2004 to 2009. Journal of Midwifery & Women's Health, 59, 1, 17-27. https://doi.org/10.1111/jmwh.12172

54.   Midwives Alliance of North America. (n.d.). *What is a midwife?* Retrieved from https://mana.org/about-midwives/what-is-a-midwife

55.   Midwives Alliance of North America. (n.d.). *The midwives model of care.* Retrieved from https://mana.org/about-midwives/midwifery-model

56.   Midwives Alliance of North America. (n.d.). *The midwives model of care.* Retrieved from https://mana.org/about-midwives/midwifery-model

57.   American College of Nurse-Midwives. (2012). *Midwifery: Evidence-based practice.* Retrieved from http://www.midwife.org/acnm/files/cclibraryfiles/filename/000000002128/midwifery%20evidence-based%20practice%20issue%20brief%20finalmay%202012.pdf

58.   American College of Nurse-Midwives. (n.d.). *Comparison of Certified Nurse-Midwives, Certified Midwives, Certified Professional Midwives clarifying the distinctions among professional midwifery credentials in the U.S.* Retrieved from http://www.midwife.org/acnm/files/ccLibrary-Files/FILENAME/000000006807/FINAL-ComparisonChart-Oct2017.pdf

59.   North American Registry of Midwives. (n.d.). *How to become a CPM.* Retrieved from http://narm.org/certification/how-to-become-a-cpm/

60.   North American Registry of Midwives. (2019). *Candidate information booklet.* Retrieved from http://narm.org/pdffiles/CIB.pdf

61.   MacDorman, M., Mathews, T.J., & Declercq, E. (2012). Home births in the United States, 1990-2009. *Centers for Disease Control and Prevention.* Retrieved from https://www.cdc.gov/nchs/data/databriefs/db84.pdf

62.   Martin, J., Hamilton, B., Osterman, M., Curtin, S., & Mathews, T.J. (2013, December 30). Births: Final data for 2012. *Centers for Disease Control and Prevention.* Retrieved from https://www.cdc.gov/nchs/data/nvsr/nvsr62/nvsr62_09.pdf

63. Centers for Disease Control and Prevention. (2018, January 31). Births: Final data for 2016. *National Vital Statistics Reports, 67, 1.* Retrieved from https://www.cdc.gov/nchs/data/nvsr/nvsr67/nvsr67_01_tables.pdf

64. Centers for Disease Control and Prevention. (n.d.). *National Vital Statistics Reports.* Retrieved from https://www.cdc.gov/nchs/products/nvsr.htm

65. Centers for Disease Control and Prevention. (2018, November 7). Births: Final data for 2017. *National Vital Statistics Reports, 67, 8.* Retrieved from https://www.cdc.gov/nchs/data/nvsr/nvsr67/nvsr67_08_tables-508.pdf

66. Centers for Disease Control and Prevention. (2011). *User guide to the 2011 natality public use file.* Retrieved from ftp://ftp.cdc.gov/pub/Health_Statistics/NCHS/Dataset_Documentation/DVS/natality/UserGuide2011.pdf

67. Kentucky Office of Vital Statistics. (n.d.). *Births by place* [Data file].

68. Midwives Alliance of North America. (n.d.). *Homebirth and community midwifery.* Retrieved from https://mana.org/about-midwives/homebirth

69. Boucher, D., Bennett, C., McFarlin, B., & Freeze, R. (2009). Staying home to give birth: Why women in the United States choose home birth. *Journal of Midwifery & Women's Health, 54, 2,* 119-126. Retrieved from https://www.medscape.com/viewarticle/589062

70. Margulis, J. (2016, May 19). What if home birth is actually safer than hospital birth? *Reset.Me.* Retrieved from http://reset.me/story/what-if-home-birth-is-actually-safer-than-hospital-birth/

71. Midwives Alliance of North America. (2012). *Homebirth position paper.* Retrieved from https://mana.org/sites/default/files/pdfs/MANAHomebirthPositionPaper_0.pdf

72. Cheyney, M., Bovbjerg, M., Everson, C., Gordon, W., Hannibal, D., & Vedam, S. (2014, January 30). Outcomes of care for 16,924 planned home births in the United States: The Midwives Alliance of North America Statistics Project, 2004 to 2009. Journal of Midwifery & Women's Health, 59, 1, 17-27. https://doi.org/10.1111/jmwh.12172

73.   Centers for Disease Control and Prevention. (n.d.). *National Vital Statistics Reports.* Retrieved from https://www.cdc.gov/nchs/products/nvsr.htm

74.   Rossen, L. (2018). Quarterly provisional estimates for infant mortality, 2015-Quarter 1, 2018. *National Center for Health Statistics, National Vital Statistics System, Vital Statistics Rapid Release Program.* Retrieved from https://www.cdc.gov/nchs/nvss/vsrr/infant-mortality-dashboard.htm

75.   Johnson, K.C. & Daviss, B.A. (2005, June 16). Outcomes of planned home births with certified professional midwives: Large prospective study in North America. *BMJ, 330, 1416.* https://doi.org/10.1136/bmj.330.7505.1416

76.   Birthplace in England Collaborative Group, Brocklehurst, P., Hardy, P., Hollowell, J., Linsell, L., Macfarlane, A.,...McCourt, C. (2011, November 23). Perinatal and maternal outcomes by planned place of birth for healthy women with low risk pregnancies: The Birthplace in England national prospective cohort study. *BMJ, 343.* doi:10.1136/bmj.d7400

77.   Olsen, O. (2008, June 28). Meta-analysis of the safety of home birth. Birth: Issues in Perinatal Care, 24, 1, 4-13. https://doi.org/10.1111/j.1523-536X.1997.00004.pp.x

78.   Janssen P., Saxell L., Page L., Klein M., Liston R., & Lee S. (2009, September 15). Outcomes of planned home birth with registered midwife versus planned hospital birth with midwife or physician. *CMAJ, 181, 6-7,* 377-383. doi: 10.1503/cmaj.081869

79.   Hutton, E., Cappalletti, A., Reitsma, A., Simioni, J., Horne, J., McGregor, C., Ahmed, R. (2016, March 15). Outcomes associated with planned place of birth among women with low-risk pregnancies. *CMAJ, 188, 5,* E80-90. doi: 10.1503/cmaj.150564

80.   de Jonge, A., Geerts, C., van der Goes, B., Mol, B., Buitendijk, S., & Nijhuis, J. (2015). Perinatal mortality and morbidity up to 28 days after birth among 743 070 low-risk planned home and hospital births: A cohort study based on three merged national perinatal databases. *BJOG, 122, 5,* 720-728. doi: 10.1111/1471-0528

81. American College of Obstetricians and Gynecologists. (2017). *Committee opinion: Planned home birth.* Retrieved from https://www.acog. org/Clinical-Guidance-and-Publications/Committee-Opinions/ Committee-on-Obstetric-Practice/Planned-Home-Birth

82. American College of Nurse-Midwives. (2011). *ACOG committee opinion on planned home birth: Opening the door to collaborative care.* Retrieved from http://www.midwife.org/ACNM/files/ccLibraryFiles/ Filename/000000000920/ACNM%20response%20to%20ACOG_746.pdf

83. Tessmer-Tuck, J. (n.d.). Homebirth and collaborating with midwives. *American College of Obstetricians and Gynecologists.* Retrieved from https://www.acog.org/About-ACOG/ACOG-Departments/ Patient-Safety-and-Quality-Improvement/How-I-Practice/ Homebirth-and-Collaborating-With-Midwives

84. Martin, N. (2018, February 22). A larger role for midwives could improve deficient U.S. care for mothers and babies. *ProPublica.* Retrieved from https://www.propublica.org/article/midwives-study-maternal-neonatal-care

85. Birth Place Lab. (2014). *Midwifery Integration State Scoring (MISS) system report card: Washington state.* Retrieved from https://www. birthplacelab.org/wp-content/uploads/2018/02/Washington.pdf

86. American College of Obstetricians and Gynecologists. (2017). *Committee opinion: Planned home birth.* Retrieved from https://www.acog. org/Clinical-Guidance-and-Publications/Committee-Opinions/ Committee-on-Obstetric-Practice/Planned-Home-Birth

87. American Academy of Pediatrics. (2013, April 29). *Policy statement: Planned home birth.* Retrieved from http://pediatrics.aappublications.org/ content/pediatrics/early/2013/04/24/peds.2013-0575.full.pdf

88. American College of Nurse-Midwives. (2011). *Position statement: Home birth.* Retrieved from http://www.midwife.org/ACNM/files/ ACNMLibraryData/UPLOADFILENAME/000000000251/Home%20Birth%20 Aug%202011.pdf

89. American College of Nurse-Midwives. (2015, December 16). Midwifery provision of home birth services. https://doi.org/10.1111/jmwh.12431

90. International Confederation of Midwives. (2017). *Position statement: Home birth.* Retrieved from https://www.internationalmidwives.org/assets/files/statement-files/2018/04/eng-home-birth14.pdf

91. Vedam, S., Stoll, K., MacDorman, M., Declercq, E., Cramer, R., Cheyney, M., …Fisher, T. (2018, February 21). Mapping integration of midwives across the United States: Impact on access, equity, and outcomes. *PLoS ONE 13,2.* https://doi.org/10.1371/journal.pone.0192523

92. Birth Place Lab. (2014). *Midwifery Integration State Scoring (MISS) system report card: Washington state.* Retrieved from https://www.birthplacelab.org/wp-content/uploads/2018/02/Washington.pdf

93. The Birth Place Lab. (2019). *University of British Columbia's Division of Midwifery.* Retrieved from https://www.birthplacelab.org/wp-content/uploads/2018/02/New-Mexico.pdf

94. The Birth Place Lab. (2019). *University of British Columbia's Division of Midwifery.* Retrieved from https://www.birthplacelab.org/wp-content/uploads/2018/02/Oregon.pdf

95. Home Birth Summit. (2019). *Collaboration.* Retrieved from https://www.homebirthsummit.org/resources/collaboration/

96. Washington State Perinatal Collaborative. (2014). *Smooth transitions: Enhancing the safety of planned out-of-hospital birth transfers.* Retrieved from http://nacpm.org/wp-content/uploads/2014/11/NACPM-Smooth-Transitions-Presentation-JMC.pdfhttp://nacpm.org/wp-content/uploads/2014/11/NACPM-Smooth-Transitions-Presentation-JMC.pdf

97. Kentucky Home Birth Coalition. (2015, September 10). *Is home birth legal in Kentucky?* Retrieved from https://kentuckyhomebirthcoalition.com/is-home-birth-legal-in-kentucky/

98. Kentucky General Assembly. (2018). *Senate Bill 134.* Retrieved from https://apps.legislature.ky.gov/record/18rs/sb134.html

99. Kentucky General Assembly. (2018). *SB 134: An act relating to permits for certified professional midwives.* Retrieved from https://apps.legislature.ky.gov/record/18rs/sb134/vote_history.pdf

100.   Kentucky General Assembly. (2019). *Senate Bill 84.* Retrieved from https://apps.legislature.ky.gov/record/19rs/sb84.html

www.ingramcontent.com/pod-product-compliance
Lightning Source LLC
Chambersburg PA
CBHW042249040426
42336CB00043B/3382